PROTECTING YOUR ERECTION

Ways to Prevent Erectile Dysfunction (ED)

Dr. Fredrick Kim

TABLE OF CONTENTS

INTRODUCTION

Erectile health is an essential aspect of overall well-being, influencing not only physical health but also emotional and mental well-being. A healthy erection is a sign of good cardiovascular function, proper blood flow, balanced hormones, and a strong connection between the mind and body. However, factors such as stress, poor diet, lack of exercise, and underlying health conditions can all contribute to erectile dysfunction (ED), which is the inability to achieve or maintain an erection sufficient for sexual activity.

In this guide, we'll explore the various elements that play a role in protecting and maintaining healthy erections. Whether you're experiencing occasional issues or want to improve your sexual health as a preventive measure, understanding the factors that influence erectile function can help you take control of your sexual health and improve your quality of life.

The key to long-term erectile health lies in a holistic approach—one that combines a balanced diet, regular physical activity, mental well-being, and healthy lifestyle choices. These efforts not only support your ability to maintain an erection but also improve your general health and vitality.

In this book, we will delve into:

The physiological mechanisms behind an erection, so you can understand what happens in your body.
How nutrition, exercise, sleep, and stress management impact erectile function.
Practical steps you can take today to protect your erections and improve your sexual health.
How to recognize early signs of erectile dysfunction and when to seek professional help.
Ultimately, this guide is designed to help you maintain a healthy and fulfilling sex life. By taking proactive steps, you can protect your erections and enjoy the benefits of optimal sexual health for years to come.

CHAPTER 1
The Physiology of an Erection

To understand how to protect and maintain healthy erections, it's essential to first grasp the basic physiology of how an erection occurs. An erection is a complex process involving the nervous system, blood vessels, hormones, and psychological factors working in harmony.

How Erections Work

Stimulus and Signal Transmission

Erections typically begin with physical or psychological stimulation. This can include touch, visual arousal, thoughts, or emotions.

The Role of the Brain: The brain processes these stimuli and sends signals down the spinal cord to the pelvic nerves.

Neurotransmitters at Play: Nitric oxide (NO) is released in the nerve endings, which triggers the dilation of blood vessels in the penis.

Blood Flow Dynamics

Arterial Blood Flow: The release of nitric oxide relaxes the smooth muscles in the arteries of the penis, allowing more blood to flow into the corpora cavernosa—two sponge-like structures in the shaft of the penis.

Engorgement and Pressure: As the corpora cavernosa fill with blood, they expand, causing the penis to become rigid. The tunica albuginea, a fibrous membrane surrounding the corpora cavernosa, traps the blood inside to maintain the erection.

Venous Restriction

During an erection, veins that normally drain blood from the penis are compressed, further helping to sustain the erection by preventing blood from flowing out.

Hormonal Support

Testosterone's Role: The hormone testosterone plays a vital role in sexual desire (libido) and erectile function. It influences the responsiveness of the brain and nerve signals involved in achieving an erection.

The Role of the Parasympathetic and Sympathetic Nervous Systems

Parasympathetic Activation: Initiates and maintains erections by promoting blood vessel relaxation.
Sympathetic Activation: Predominantly responsible for ejaculation and the resolution phase of the erection.

Key Factors Affecting Erectile Function

Blood Vessel Health

Healthy blood vessels are critical for sufficient blood flow. Conditions such as atherosclerosis or hypertension can impair this process.

Nervous System Function
Damage to the nerves that send signals to the penis—due to diabetes, surgery, or injury—can lead to erectile dysfunction.

Hormonal Balance
Low testosterone levels or hormonal imbalances can interfere with sexual desire and the physiological process of an erection.

Psychological Factors
Anxiety, stress, depression, and relationship issues can inhibit the brain's ability to send the right signals to initiate an erection.

Erection Types
Reflexogenic Erections
Triggered by direct physical contact with the penis or nearby areas.

Psychogenic Erections
Initiated by erotic thoughts, sights, sounds, or fantasies.

Nocturnal Erections

Spontaneous erections that occur during REM (rapid eye movement) sleep, indicating healthy erectile function.

Understanding the physiology of an erection lays the groundwork for recognizing and addressing potential issues. A healthy erection depends on proper blood flow, efficient nerve function, balanced hormones, and a supportive psychological state. The chapters that follow will dive deeper into how lifestyle, nutrition, and other factors influence these components, empowering you to take proactive steps to protect your erection health.

CHAPTER 2
The Role of Diet in Erectile Health

What you eat plays a crucial role in maintaining erectile function. A healthy diet supports blood circulation, hormone production, and overall vascular health—all essential factors for achieving and sustaining erections.

How Diet Affects Erectile Function

Blood Circulation
Erections depend on adequate blood flow to the penis. Foods that promote cardiovascular health also enhance blood circulation, benefiting erectile function.

Hormone Production
Key nutrients are essential for the production of testosterone and other hormones critical to sexual health.

Inflammation and Oxidative Stress
Poor dietary choices can lead to chronic inflammation and oxidative stress, damaging blood vessels and impairing erectile function.

Weight Management

A healthy diet helps maintain a healthy weight, reducing the risk of obesity—a significant contributor to erectile dysfunction (ED).

Nutrients Essential for Erectile Health
Nitric Oxide Boosters
Nitric oxide (NO) is vital for relaxing blood vessels and enhancing blood flow. Foods rich in nitrates can help increase NO levels.
Examples: Beets, spinach, arugula, celery.

Antioxidants
Antioxidants combat oxidative stress, protecting blood vessels and improving vascular health.
Examples: Berries, dark chocolate, green tea.

Zinc
Zinc supports testosterone production and overall sexual health.
Examples: Oysters, pumpkin seeds, chickpeas.

Vitamin D
Low vitamin D levels are associated with ED. This vitamin supports testosterone levels and vascular function.
Examples: Salmon, fortified foods, sunlight exposure.

Omega-3 Fatty Acids
Omega-3s improve heart health, reduce inflammation, and enhance circulation.

Examples: Fatty fish (salmon, mackerel), flaxseeds, walnuts.

L-Arginine
An amino acid that helps produce nitric oxide and improve blood flow.
Examples: Nuts, seeds, poultry.

Foods to Include for Erectile Health
Fruits and Vegetables
Citrus Fruits: Rich in vitamin C and flavonoids, improving blood flow.
Leafy Greens: High in nitrates and antioxidants.

Whole Grains
Improve heart health and reduce the risk of conditions like diabetes that can affect erections.

Healthy Fats
Avocado, Olive Oil, Nuts: Provide heart-healthy fats that support circulation and hormone production.

Lean Proteins
Chicken, Turkey, Fish: Offer essential amino acids for blood vessel health.

Dark Chocolate
Contains flavonoids that boost circulation.

Green Tea

Packed with antioxidants that promote vascular health.

Foods to Avoid
Processed Foods
High in unhealthy fats, sodium, and sugar, leading to poor cardiovascular health.

Sugary Beverages
Can lead to obesity and diabetes, both of which are linked to ED.

Trans Fats
Found in fried and processed foods, trans fats contribute to arterial damage and reduced blood flow.

Excessive Alcohol
While moderate alcohol consumption may be okay, excessive drinking can impair erectile function.

Sample Erectile-Health Meal Plan
Breakfast:
Spinach and mushroom omelet with whole-grain toast.
A glass of fresh orange juice.

Lunch:
Grilled salmon salad with arugula, walnuts, and a lemon-olive oil dressing.

A side of quinoa.

Snack:
Handful of mixed berries and a few dark chocolate pieces.

Dinner:
Baked chicken breast with roasted sweet potatoes and steamed broccoli.

A cup of green tea.

The Role of Hydration
Staying well-hydrated is essential for overall health and can also benefit erectile function. Water supports blood circulation and reduces the risk of fatigue or sluggishness that might impact sexual performance.

A diet rich in whole, nutrient-dense foods can significantly enhance erectile health by improving blood flow, supporting hormone production, and reducing the risk of chronic diseases. By making informed dietary choices, you can take a proactive step toward protecting your erections and enjoying a healthier, more fulfilling sex life.

CHAPTER 3
Exercise and Erectile Function

Exercise plays a vital role in maintaining erectile health by improving blood flow, boosting testosterone levels, and supporting overall physical and mental well-being. A sedentary lifestyle, on the other hand, can lead to obesity, poor circulation, and cardiovascular issues, all of which are common contributors to erectile dysfunction (ED).

The Link Between Exercise and Erectile Function

Improved Cardiovascular Health

Erections rely on healthy blood flow, and exercise strengthens the heart and arteries, improving circulation.

Regular aerobic activities, like walking or swimming, reduce the risk of conditions such as hypertension and atherosclerosis, which impair blood flow to the penis.

Hormonal Benefits

Physical activity boosts testosterone levels, a critical hormone for sexual desire and erectile health.

Weight Management

Exercise helps prevent obesity, a major risk factor for ED, by reducing excess fat and maintaining a healthy body mass index (BMI).

Mental Health Improvements
Regular exercise reduces stress, anxiety, and depression, all of which can negatively affect erectile function.

Strengthened Pelvic Floor Muscles
Targeted exercises improve the strength of the pelvic floor muscles, enhancing blood flow to the genital area and supporting sustained erections.
Best Types of Exercise for Erectile Health

Aerobic Exercises
Improve cardiovascular health and overall circulation.
Examples:
Brisk walking
Running or jogging
Swimming
Cycling

Strength Training
Boosts testosterone levels and supports muscle mass, which can indirectly improve sexual performance.
Examples:
Weightlifting
Resistance band workouts
Bodyweight exercises (push-ups, squats)

Kegel Exercises

Specifically target the pelvic floor muscles to enhance erectile function and control.
How to Perform Kegels:
Identify the pelvic floor muscles by stopping urination midstream.
Contract these muscles for 3-5 seconds, then relax for the same amount of time.
Repeat 10-15 times, three times a day.

Yoga and Flexibility Training
Reduces stress and increases flexibility, contributing to improved sexual stamina and performance.
Poses to Try:
Downward Dog
Cobra Pose
Bridge Pose

Developing a Sustainable Exercise Routine
Start Small
Begin with 15-20 minutes of activity per day and gradually increase the intensity and duration.

Consistency is Key
Aim for at least 150 minutes of moderate-intensity aerobic exercise per week, as recommended by health professionals.

Mix It Up
Combine aerobic, strength, and flexibility exercises to target different aspects of health.

Listen to Your Body
Avoid overexertion and ensure adequate rest to prevent burnout or injury.

Make It Enjoyable
Choose activities you enjoy to increase the likelihood of sticking to your routine.

Overcoming Barriers to Exercise
Lack of Time
Incorporate shorter sessions, such as 10-minute walks after meals or quick home workouts.

Physical Limitations
Modify exercises to accommodate your fitness level or any medical conditions. Consult with a professional if needed.

Motivation Challenges
Set realistic goals and track your progress to stay motivated.

The Role of Sex as Exercise
Sex itself is a form of physical activity that can improve cardiovascular health and reduce stress. Engaging in regular sexual activity may help maintain erectile function, although it should be complemented by other forms of exercise for overall fitness.

Exercise is one of the most effective natural remedies for improving erectile function. By strengthening your cardiovascular system, enhancing testosterone levels, and reducing stress, physical activity lays the foundation for long-term sexual health. Start small, stay consistent, and make exercise an integral part of your lifestyle to enjoy both physical and sexual vitality.

CHAPTER 4
The Impact of Alcohol and Tobacco

Lifestyle choices like alcohol consumption and tobacco use have significant effects on erectile function. While occasional indulgence may seem harmless, excessive or long-term use can damage the systems that support healthy erections.

How Alcohol Affects Erectile Function

Short-Term Effects

Alcohol is a depressant that can impair the nervous system, slowing down the brain's ability to send arousal signals to the penis.

Excessive drinking can lead to "whiskey dick," a temporary inability to achieve or maintain an erection.

Long-Term Effects

Chronic alcohol abuse damages the liver, leading to hormonal imbalances.

The liver processes testosterone; alcohol impairs this function, leading to lower testosterone levels.

Excessive alcohol consumption can cause nerve damage (neuropathy), including the nerves involved in erectile function.

Alcohol contributes to cardiovascular issues like high blood pressure, which restrict blood flow to the penis.

Dehydration and Blood Flow
Alcohol dehydrates the body, reducing blood volume and potentially impairing circulation necessary for erections.

Psychological Impact
Long-term alcohol abuse is linked to anxiety, depression, and reduced libido, all of which negatively affect sexual performance.
How Tobacco Affects Erectile Function

Impact on Blood Flow
Tobacco contains nicotine, a vasoconstrictor that narrows blood vessels and restricts blood flow to the penis.
Smoking damages the endothelial lining of blood vessels, reducing nitric oxide production, which is essential for erections.

Cardiovascular Damage
Long-term smoking increases the risk of atherosclerosis (plaque buildup in arteries), further impeding blood flow.

Hormonal Disruption
Smoking lowers testosterone levels and increases cortisol, a stress hormone that can negatively affect erectile health.

Oxidative Stress and Inflammation

Tobacco introduces toxins and free radicals into the body, causing oxidative stress and chronic inflammation, both of which impair erectile function.

Secondhand Smoke
Even exposure to secondhand smoke can have similar negative effects on vascular health and erectile function.

Combined Effects of Alcohol and Tobacco
When used together, alcohol and tobacco amplify their harmful effects. For example:

Alcohol and tobacco together increase oxidative stress and damage blood vessels more than either substance alone.
Chronic use of both substances is strongly linked to severe erectile dysfunction, often requiring medical intervention.

Practical Steps to Minimize Impact
Moderate Alcohol Consumption
Follow recommended guidelines: no more than two drinks per day for men.
Opt for lower-alcohol beverages like wine, which may offer some cardiovascular benefits in moderation.
Stay hydrated while drinking to reduce dehydration-related effects.

Quit Smoking

Seek professional help or support groups to quit smoking.
Consider nicotine replacement therapy or medications to ease withdrawal symptoms.
Explore behavioral therapy to address psychological triggers for smoking.

Adopt a Healthier Lifestyle
Replace drinking and smoking habits with healthier alternatives, like exercise or hobbies.
Build a support network to encourage and sustain these lifestyle changes.

Regular Check-Ups
Consult a healthcare provider for tests on vascular and hormonal health, especially if alcohol or tobacco use has been prolonged.

Benefits of Cutting Back or Quitting
Improved Circulation
Quitting smoking or reducing alcohol intake can restore healthy blood flow within weeks.

Boosted Testosterone Levels
Testosterone production improves, enhancing libido and erectile function.

Better Overall Health
Reducing alcohol and tobacco use lowers the risk of chronic conditions like heart disease, diabetes, and high blood pressure.

Enhanced Psychological Well-Being
Cutting back on these substances can reduce stress, anxiety, and depression, leading to better sexual performance.

While occasional, moderate alcohol consumption may not significantly harm erectile health, excessive drinking and smoking can have severe, long-lasting effects. Protecting your erections means making informed choices about alcohol and tobacco use. By minimizing or eliminating these habits, you can improve your overall health, restore optimal erectile function, and enjoy a better quality of life.

CHAPTER 5

Managing Stress and Mental Health

Mental health plays a critical role in maintaining erectile function. Stress, anxiety, depression, and other psychological factors can disrupt the delicate balance of hormones and neural signals necessary for achieving and sustaining an erection.

The Connection Between Mental Health and Erectile Function

Stress and Erectile Dysfunction (ED)

Stress activates the body's fight-or-flight response, releasing cortisol and adrenaline, which can restrict blood flow to the penis.

Chronic stress disrupts the balance of hormones, lowering testosterone levels and impairing libido.

Anxiety and Performance Pressure

Fear of failure or performance anxiety can create a vicious cycle where worry about erectile difficulties leads to more dysfunction.

Social and relationship pressures can amplify anxiety and negatively impact sexual confidence.

Depression

Depression reduces libido and interferes with brain signaling required for arousal.

Some antidepressant medications, particularly selective serotonin reuptake inhibitors (SSRIs), can contribute to ED as a side effect.

Emotional Well-Being and Sexual Desire
Positive mental health fosters better communication and intimacy, which are vital for a satisfying sexual experience.

How Stress Impacts the Body
Hormonal Effects: Chronic stress increases cortisol levels, which suppress testosterone and other hormones needed for sexual health.
Physical Effects: Prolonged stress can lead to high blood pressure, cardiovascular problems, and fatigue, all of which negatively affect erectile function.
Behavioral Effects: Stress often leads to unhealthy habits like overeating, drinking, or smoking, compounding its effects on ED.

Strategies to Manage Stress and Improve Mental Health
Mindfulness and Meditation
Practice Mindfulness: Focus on the present moment to reduce anxiety and improve emotional regulation.
Meditation Techniques: Deep breathing, guided imagery, or progressive muscle relaxation can help calm the mind.

Regular Exercise
Physical activity reduces cortisol and increases endorphins, improving mood and reducing stress. Activities like yoga or tai chi are particularly effective for managing stress.

Therapy and Counseling
Cognitive Behavioral Therapy (CBT): Helps identify and challenge negative thought patterns contributing to ED.
Couples Therapy: Improves communication and addresses relationship issues that may be causing stress.

Time Management
Organize your day to avoid feeling overwhelmed. Prioritize tasks and take breaks to recharge.

Sleep Hygiene
Adequate sleep regulates cortisol and supports healthy testosterone production.
Maintain a consistent sleep schedule and create a relaxing bedtime routine.

Social Connections
Engage with friends, family, or support groups to share experiences and reduce feelings of isolation.

Relaxation Techniques
Activities like journaling, art, or spending time in nature can help reduce stress.

Limit Stressors
Identify and reduce unnecessary stressors in your life, whether it's overcommitment or toxic relationships.

When to Seek Professional Help
Persistent feelings of anxiety, depression, or stress that interfere with daily life or sexual function.
Difficulty managing emotions or coping with stress despite trying self-help strategies.
Signs of a mental health disorder, such as mood swings, loss of interest in activities, or significant changes in appetite or sleep.

Natural Remedies to Support Mental Health
Herbal Supplements
Ashwagandha: Helps lower cortisol levels and improve stress resilience.
Valerian Root: Promotes relaxation and better sleep.

Dietary Choices
Foods rich in magnesium (e.g., spinach, almonds) and omega-3 fatty acids (e.g., salmon, walnuts) support brain health and reduce stress.

The Importance of Intimacy
Building emotional intimacy with a partner can alleviate stress and enhance sexual confidence. Open communication about fears, desires, and

expectations strengthens trust and can help address erectile difficulties together.

Managing stress and mental health is essential for protecting erectile function and maintaining a healthy sex life. By adopting effective stress-reduction techniques, seeking professional help when needed, and fostering emotional well-being, you can break the cycle of stress-induced erectile dysfunction and achieve greater overall health and satisfaction.

CHAPTER 6
Sleep and Hormonal Balance

Sleep is a cornerstone of overall health, including sexual health. Adequate, high-quality sleep helps regulate hormones essential for libido and erectile function. Poor sleep patterns, whether due to insomnia, sleep apnea, or irregular schedules, can disrupt hormonal balance, leading to erectile dysfunction (ED) and diminished sexual performance.

The Role of Sleep in Hormonal Balance

Testosterone Production
The majority of testosterone is produced during deep sleep, particularly in the REM (Rapid Eye Movement) phase.
Poor sleep reduces testosterone levels, directly impacting libido and erectile function.

Cortisol Regulation
Chronic sleep deprivation elevates cortisol, a stress hormone that suppresses testosterone production and impairs erections.

Growth Hormone (GH)
GH, released during deep sleep, aids in tissue repair and overall vitality, supporting physical stamina and sexual health.

Other Hormones
Leptin and ghrelin, which regulate appetite, can become imbalanced with poor sleep, contributing to weight gain and obesity—key risk factors for ED.
Effects of Poor Sleep on Erectile Function

Reduced Libido
Sleep deprivation leads to fatigue and low energy, reducing sexual desire.

Impaired Nitric Oxide Production
Sleep disruption impairs the body's ability to produce nitric oxide, essential for blood vessel relaxation and healthy erections.

Increased Risk of Chronic Conditions
Sleep disorders are associated with hypertension, diabetes, and obesity, which significantly increase the risk of ED.

Mental Health Impact
Poor sleep exacerbates stress, anxiety, and depression, all of which contribute to erectile dysfunction.
Common Sleep Disorders and Their Impact on Erectile Health

Sleep Apnea

A condition where breathing stops temporarily during sleep, reducing oxygen levels and testosterone production.
Strongly associated with cardiovascular issues that impair blood flow to the penis.

Insomnia
Chronic difficulty falling or staying asleep leads to hormonal imbalances and mental fatigue.

Shift Work Sleep Disorder
Irregular work hours disrupt the body's natural circadian rhythm, impairing hormone production.
Optimizing Sleep for Better Hormonal Health

Establish a Sleep Routine
Go to bed and wake up at the same time each day to regulate your internal clock.

Create a Sleep-Friendly Environment
Keep your bedroom cool, dark, and quiet.
Invest in a comfortable mattress and pillows.

Limit Stimulants
Avoid caffeine, nicotine, and heavy meals within a few hours of bedtime.
Reduce alcohol consumption, which disrupts REM sleep.

Reduce Screen Time

Minimize exposure to blue light from phones, tablets, and computers at least an hour before bed.

Incorporate Relaxation Techniques
Practice meditation, deep breathing, or light yoga to unwind before bed.

Exercise Regularly
Regular physical activity improves sleep quality but avoid vigorous workouts close to bedtime.

Seek Treatment for Sleep Disorders
If you suspect sleep apnea or chronic insomnia, consult a healthcare professional for diagnosis and treatment.

Natural Supplements for Better Sleep
Melatonin
A natural hormone that regulates sleep-wake cycles.

Magnesium
Helps relax muscles and calm the nervous system.

Valerian Root
A herbal remedy known for promoting relaxation and sleep.

Chamomile
Often used as a tea, chamomile has calming effects that aid sleep.

Sample Evening Routine for Optimal Sleep and Hormonal Balance

6:00 PM: Eat a light, balanced dinner with minimal caffeine and sugar.

7:30 PM: Engage in a relaxing activity, such as reading or spending time with family.

8:30 PM: Dim the lights and avoid screens. Consider a warm bath to relax your body.

9:30 PM: Practice mindfulness or light stretches to calm the mind.

10:00 PM: Head to bed, aiming for 7-9 hours of sleep.

Sleep is not just a time for rest but a critical process for hormonal regulation and overall health. By prioritizing high-quality sleep and addressing any sleep-related issues, you can boost testosterone levels, reduce stress, and support your body's ability to achieve and sustain erections. A well-rested body and mind pave the way for improved sexual performance and vitality.

CHAPTER 7
Maintaining a Healthy Weight

Your weight plays a crucial role in sexual health and erectile function. Excess body weight, particularly obesity, can lead to hormonal imbalances, reduced blood flow, and increased risk of chronic conditions that contribute to erectile dysfunction (ED).

The Link Between Weight and Erectile Function

Impact on Blood Flow

Obesity contributes to atherosclerosis (narrowing of blood vessels), which restricts blood flow to the penis, making it difficult to achieve or sustain an erection.

Hormonal Imbalances

Excess fat tissue converts testosterone to estrogen, reducing testosterone levels essential for libido and erectile health.

Obesity is associated with insulin resistance, which can lead to lower testosterone levels.

Increased Risk of Chronic Conditions

Obesity increases the risk of type 2 diabetes, high blood pressure, and heart disease, all of which are significant contributors to ED.

Inflammation and Oxidative Stress

Excess weight leads to chronic inflammation and oxidative stress, damaging blood vessels and impairing erectile function.

Mental Health Implications
Being overweight can affect self-esteem and lead to depression and anxiety, which can exacerbate ED.
Benefits of Maintaining a Healthy Weight

Improved Blood Flow
Reduced body fat helps maintain healthy blood vessels, improving circulation to the penis.

Enhanced Hormonal Balance
Weight loss can restore testosterone levels, improving libido and sexual performance.

Lower Risk of Chronic Diseases
Achieving a healthy weight reduces the likelihood of diabetes, hypertension, and heart disease.

Boosted Energy Levels
Carrying less weight improves stamina and physical endurance, enhancing overall vitality and sexual performance.

Better Mental Health
Weight loss often leads to improved confidence, reduced stress, and a more positive body image.
Strategies for Achieving and Maintaining a Healthy Weight

Adopt a Balanced Diet
Focus on Whole Foods: Prioritize fruits, vegetables, lean proteins, whole grains, and healthy fats.
Limit Processed Foods: Avoid excessive sugar, refined carbs, and unhealthy fats that contribute to weight gain.
Portion Control: Use smaller plates and listen to your body's hunger cues.

Incorporate Regular Exercise
Aerobic Activities: Walking, running, cycling, or swimming improve cardiovascular health and burn calories.
Strength Training: Build muscle, which boosts metabolism and supports long-term weight management.
Consistency: Aim for at least 150 minutes of moderate-intensity exercise per week.

Set Realistic Goals
Focus on gradual, sustainable weight loss of 1-2 pounds per week.

Track Your Progress
Use apps or journals to monitor your food intake, exercise, and weight changes.

Stay Hydrated
Drink plenty of water to support metabolism and reduce unnecessary calorie intake.

Prioritize Sleep
Poor sleep is linked to weight gain; ensure you get 7-9 hours of quality sleep each night.

Seek Support
Work with a nutritionist, trainer, or support group to stay motivated and accountable.

Overcoming Barriers to Weight Loss

Lack of Time
Integrate small changes like taking stairs, meal prepping, or short exercise sessions into your routine.

Emotional Eating
Address triggers like stress or boredom by practicing mindfulness or seeking therapy if needed.

Plateaus
Adjust your diet or workout routine if weight loss stalls; sometimes, the body needs a new stimulus.

Dietary Tips to Boost Erectile Health

Eat Foods Rich in Antioxidants
Examples: Berries, spinach, nuts, and dark chocolate improve blood flow and reduce inflammation.

Increase Omega-3 Fatty Acids

Examples: Salmon, walnuts, and flaxseeds support cardiovascular health.

Include Foods High in Zinc
Examples: Shellfish, pumpkin seeds, and lean meats help maintain testosterone levels.

Limit Alcohol and Sugary Beverages
These contribute to weight gain and impair sexual function.

The Role of Medical Interventions
Consult a Healthcare Provider
Seek guidance for underlying conditions, like thyroid issues or metabolic disorders, that may hinder weight loss.

Consider Bariatric Surgery
For severe obesity, weight-loss surgery may improve erectile function by addressing both physical and hormonal factors.

Medications
Discuss options for appetite suppression or metabolic support if lifestyle changes alone aren't effective.
Maintaining a healthy weight is one of the most effective ways to protect and improve erectile health. By adopting a balanced diet, engaging in regular physical activity, and addressing underlying barriers to weight loss, you can achieve a healthier body and

a more satisfying sex life. Weight management not only enhances your physical appearance but also supports the hormonal and vascular systems critical for sexual vitality.

CHAPTER 8
Understanding and Avoiding Medications That Affect Erections

Certain medications can interfere with your ability to achieve or maintain an erection. While many drugs are essential for treating medical conditions, they may have side effects that negatively impact sexual function.

How Medications Affect Erectile Function

Hormonal Disruption

Some medications lower testosterone levels or disrupt the balance of other hormones critical for erectile health.

Impaired Blood Flow

Drugs that constrict blood vessels or reduce blood pressure can limit blood flow to the penis, affecting erections.

Neurological Effects

Medications that alter brain chemistry can interfere with arousal, libido, and the neural signals needed for an erection.

Psychological Impact

Side effects like fatigue, mood changes, or anxiety can indirectly reduce sexual desire and performance.

Common Medications That Can Affect Erections
Antihypertensives (Blood Pressure Medications)
Examples: Beta-blockers (e.g., metoprolol), diuretics (e.g., hydrochlorothiazide).
Impact: Reduce blood pressure but may also decrease blood flow to the penis.

Antidepressants and Antipsychotics
Examples: SSRIs (e.g., sertraline, fluoxetine), tricyclics (e.g., amitriptyline), antipsychotics (e.g., risperidone).

Impact: Alter brain chemistry, potentially lowering libido and impairing erectile function.

Opioids and Pain Relievers
Examples: Morphine, oxycodone.
Impact: Suppress testosterone production and reduce sexual desire.

Antiandrogens and Hormone Therapies
Examples: Medications for prostate cancer (e.g., leuprolide), treatments for hormone-sensitive conditions.
Impact: Directly lower testosterone levels.

Sedatives and Sleep Aids

Examples: Benzodiazepines (e.g., diazepam), sleep medications (e.g., zolpidem).
Impact: Depress the central nervous system, reducing libido and arousal.

Chemotherapy and Cancer Treatments
Examples: Certain chemotherapeutic agents, radiation therapy near the pelvic area.
Impact: Damage to blood vessels and nerves essential for erections.

Antihistamines and Decongestants
Examples: Diphenhydramine, pseudoephedrine.
Impact: Temporary reduction in blood flow or altered nervous system activity.

Recreational Drugs
Examples: Alcohol, cocaine, marijuana.
Impact: Impair arousal and erection mechanisms through various pathways.

Strategies to Minimize Medication-Related ED
Discuss Concerns with Your Doctor
Be open about sexual side effects when prescribed a new medication.

Seek Alternatives
In some cases, a different drug with fewer sexual side effects may be available.
For example, switching from a beta-blocker to an ACE inhibitor may preserve erectile function.

Adjust Dosages
Lowering the dose of certain medications may reduce their impact on sexual health.

Timing Adjustments
Taking medications at different times may help minimize their interference with sexual activity.

Monitor Testosterone Levels
If a medication reduces testosterone, discuss supplementation or alternatives with your doctor.

Address Underlying Conditions
Treating the root cause of a condition (e.g., high blood pressure or depression) may reduce the need for medications that impact erectile function.

Lifestyle Changes to Counteract Medication Effects

Diet and Exercise
Maintaining a healthy lifestyle can reduce dependency on medications for conditions like hypertension or diabetes.

Stress Management
Lowering stress through mindfulness or therapy may reduce the need for anxiety or depression medications.

Weight Management

Losing weight may improve conditions like sleep apnea or metabolic syndrome, reducing the need for medication.

When to Consider Additional Treatments
Erectile Dysfunction Medications
Examples: Sildenafil (Viagra), tadalafil (Cialis).
Purpose: Can counteract ED caused by necessary medications under a doctor's guidance.

Vacuum Erection Devices
Non-invasive tools to assist with achieving erections.

Testosterone Replacement Therapy (TRT)
For those with low testosterone due to necessary medications, TRT may help but should only be used under medical supervision.

Psychological Counseling
If ED is partly due to the psychological impact of medication side effects, therapy can help.
Important Considerations
Do Not Stop Medications Abruptly: Always consult a healthcare provider before discontinuing or changing any prescribed medication.
Monitor Side Effects: Keep track of how medications affect your sexual health and report issues promptly.
Balance Risks and Benefits: Weigh the necessity of a medication against its impact on erectile function with your doctor.

While medications are sometimes necessary for managing chronic conditions, their impact on erectile health should not be ignored. By understanding the potential side effects, working closely with your healthcare provider, and making lifestyle adjustments, you can minimize the impact of medications on your sexual function while maintaining overall health.

CHAPTER 9

Strengthening Pelvic Floor Muscles

The pelvic floor muscles play a crucial role in erectile function and overall sexual health. These muscles support the bladder, bowel, and sexual organs, contributing to the firmness and sustainability of erections. Strengthening the pelvic floor improves blood flow to the penis, enhances control during sexual activity, and can even help prevent erectile dysfunction (ED).

The Role of Pelvic Floor Muscles in Erectile Function

Support for Blood Flow
Strong pelvic muscles help trap blood in the penis during an erection, maintaining rigidity.

Improved Ejaculatory Control
A well-conditioned pelvic floor aids in controlling ejaculation and prolonging sexual performance.

Bladder and Bowel Health
Strengthening these muscles can reduce the risk of urinary incontinence and other pelvic issues, indirectly boosting confidence and sexual function.

Benefits of Pelvic Floor Exercises

Increased Erection Hardness

Stronger muscles improve blood flow and pressure during erections.

Enhanced Orgasm Intensity
Toned pelvic muscles contribute to more powerful and satisfying orgasms.

Reduced Risk of ED
Regular pelvic floor exercises can prevent and sometimes reverse mild erectile dysfunction.

Improved Recovery Post-Surgery
Exercises are particularly beneficial for men recovering from prostate surgery or other pelvic procedures.
How to Identify Pelvic Floor Muscles

Stopping Urine Mid-Stream
Begin to urinate and then try to stop the flow. The muscles you use are your pelvic floor muscles.

Tightening Without Involving Other Muscles
Tighten the muscles as if you're trying to prevent passing gas. Avoid using your thighs, buttocks, or abdominal muscles.

Feel for Activation
Place your fingers on the area between your scrotum and anus while contracting. You should feel a slight lifting sensation.

Effective Pelvic Floor Exercises
Kegel Exercises
How to Perform:
Contract the pelvic floor muscles for 5 seconds.
Relax for 5 seconds.
Repeat 10-15 times, 2-3 times daily.
Gradually increase the duration of contractions as your muscles strengthen.

Bridge Pose
How to Perform:
Lie on your back with knees bent and feet flat on the floor.
Lift your hips while squeezing your pelvic floor muscles.
Hold for 3-5 seconds, then lower.
Perform 10-15 repetitions daily.

Squats with Pelvic Activation
How to Perform:
Stand with feet shoulder-width apart.
Lower into a squat position while engaging the pelvic floor.
Return to standing, maintaining the muscle contraction.
Perform 10 repetitions.

Pelvic Tilts
How to Perform:
Lie on your back with knees bent.

Flatten your lower back against the floor by tightening your abdominal and pelvic muscles.
Hold for 5 seconds, then release.
Repeat 10-15 times.

Heel Slides with Contraction
How to Perform:
Lie on your back with one knee bent and the other leg straight.
Slide the heel of the straight leg towards your buttock while engaging the pelvic floor.
Slide back to the starting position.
Perform 10 repetitions on each side.

Tips for Effective Training
Consistency is Key
Perform pelvic floor exercises daily for noticeable results.

Focus on Proper Technique
Avoid holding your breath or using other muscles during the exercises.

Be Patient
It may take 4-6 weeks of regular practice to see improvements in erectile function.

Combine with Other Healthy Habits
Exercise, diet, and stress management complement pelvic floor training.

Seek Professional Guidance
A physical therapist specializing in men's health can provide personalized guidance if needed.

Common Mistakes to Avoid
Overtraining
Excessive exercise can lead to muscle fatigue and worsen symptoms.

Ignoring Adjacent Muscles
While focusing on the pelvic floor, maintain overall core strength for better support.

Irregular Practice
Inconsistent exercise will not yield the desired results.

Expecting Immediate Results
Improvements take time and consistent effort.

Strengthening your pelvic floor muscles is a simple yet highly effective way to improve erectile function and overall sexual health. Regularly performing these exercises can lead to harder erections, better control, and increased confidence. Whether as a preventative measure or part of a comprehensive approach to managing ED, pelvic floor training is a powerful tool for enhancing your intimate life.

CHAPTER 10

Routine Check-ups and Professional Guidance

Regular medical check-ups and seeking professional advice are essential for maintaining erectile health and overall well-being. Many underlying health issues, such as cardiovascular disease, diabetes, and hormonal imbalances, can manifest as erectile dysfunction (ED). Early detection and proactive management of these conditions can improve your quality of life and protect your sexual health.

Why Routine Check-ups Matter

Early Detection of Underlying Conditions
ED can be an early warning sign of serious health problems, such as heart disease or diabetes.

Monitoring Hormonal Levels
Regular testing can identify imbalances in testosterone or other hormones critical for sexual health.

Tracking Cardiovascular Health
Checking blood pressure, cholesterol, and vascular health ensures proper blood flow, which is crucial for erections.

Preventive Care

Routine visits help catch potential problems before they develop into serious issues.

Customized Treatment Plans
Your doctor can tailor recommendations based on your unique medical history and lifestyle.

What to Expect During a Check-Up
Medical History Review
Your doctor will ask about your overall health, medications, lifestyle, and any symptoms of ED.

Physical Examination
Includes checking the heart, blood pressure, and genitals to rule out physical causes.

Lab Tests
Common Tests Include:
Blood Tests: Evaluate cholesterol, blood sugar, and hormone levels.
Urine Tests: Check for diabetes or infections.
Liver and Kidney Function Tests: Ensure metabolic health.

Specialized Assessments
Penile Doppler Ultrasound: Measures blood flow to the penis.
Nocturnal Penile Tumescence Test: Assesses erections during sleep to determine psychological vs. physical causes.

Mental Health Evaluation
Screening for depression, anxiety, or stress-related issues that could impact sexual function.

When to Seek Professional Guidance
Persistent ED Symptoms
If erection difficulties occur regularly, consult a doctor to identify the root cause.

Sudden Onset of ED
Abrupt changes in erectile function may signal serious medical issues requiring immediate attention.

Associated Symptoms
Seek help if ED is accompanied by fatigue, weight changes, or reduced libido.

Unresponsive to Lifestyle Changes
If improvements in diet, exercise, or stress management don't resolve ED, professional guidance is necessary.

Concerns About Medications
Discuss alternative treatments if medications are causing sexual side effects.

Types of Professionals to Consult
Primary Care Physician (PCP)
Initial point of contact for routine health assessments and general advice.

Urologist
Specialist in male reproductive health and urinary
tract issues.

Endocrinologist
Expert in hormonal imbalances and conditions like
low testosterone or thyroid disorders.

Cardiologist
For cases where ED may be linked to heart or
vascular health.

Psychologist or Counselor
Address psychological factors such as anxiety,
depression, or relationship issues.

Pelvic Floor Physical Therapist
Guides in strengthening muscles that support
erectile function.

Benefits of Professional Guidance
Accurate Diagnosis
Professionals use advanced tools and tests to
pinpoint the exact cause of ED.

Access to Treatment Options
From medications and therapy to surgical solutions,
doctors can recommend the best approach.

Comprehensive Health Improvement

Addressing ED often leads to better overall health outcomes, such as improved heart and metabolic health.

Emotional Support
Talking to an expert helps alleviate anxiety and provides clarity about your condition.

Ongoing Monitoring
Regular follow-ups ensure treatments are effective and adjusted as needed.

Questions to Ask Your Doctor
What could be causing my erectile issues?
What tests should I undergo to diagnose the problem?
Are there medications or treatments that can help?
How do lifestyle changes impact my condition?
Could my current medications be contributing to ED?
Are there risks associated with treatment options?

Proactive Steps Before Your Appointment
Track Symptoms
Note frequency, duration, and severity of erectile issues.

List Medications
Include prescriptions, over-the-counter drugs, and supplements.

Assess Lifestyle Factors
Document diet, exercise, stress levels, and sleep patterns.

Prepare Questions
Write down concerns to ensure they are addressed during your visit.

Routine check-ups and professional guidance are vital for diagnosing and managing erectile dysfunction effectively. These visits not only help preserve sexual health but also ensure overall well-being. By collaborating with healthcare providers, you can address underlying causes, explore treatment options, and regain confidence in your sexual performance. Don't wait—proactive care is the key to protecting your health and vitality.

CHAPTER 11
Natural Remedies and Lifestyle Changes

When it comes to improving erectile function, natural remedies and lifestyle changes can often provide effective results. These approaches focus on optimizing overall health and addressing the underlying factors that may contribute to erectile dysfunction (ED). Whether used alone or in conjunction with medical treatments, natural methods can play a crucial role in enhancing sexual performance and overall well-being.

The Role of Lifestyle in Erectile Health

Many aspects of daily life can impact erectile function, including diet, exercise, stress, and sleep. By adopting healthy habits and making specific lifestyle changes, you can enhance blood flow, reduce stress, and maintain hormonal balance, all of which contribute to better erectile function.

Diet and Nutrition

A balanced, nutrient-rich diet plays a vital role in erectile health by supporting cardiovascular function and hormonal balance.

Foods That Promote Erectile Health:
Leafy Greens: High in nitrates, which help improve blood flow (e.g., spinach, kale).

Beets: Contain natural nitrates that help dilate blood vessels and improve circulation.

Oily Fish: Rich in omega-3 fatty acids, which improve cardiovascular health (e.g., salmon, mackerel).

Nuts and Seeds: Provide essential fatty acids and antioxidants for heart health (e.g., almonds, walnuts).

Berries: Packed with flavonoids, which promote circulation and reduce inflammation.

Garlic: Known to support blood flow by promoting nitric oxide production in the body.

Avoid or Limit:

Excess Sugar and Refined Carbs: Can contribute to insulin resistance and poor blood circulation.

Processed Foods: High in unhealthy fats, which can clog arteries and impair blood flow.

Excessive Alcohol: Can decrease testosterone levels and impair erectile function.

Regular Physical Activity

Exercise is one of the most powerful ways to boost erectile function. Physical activity helps improve blood flow, reduce stress, and support overall health, which can directly enhance sexual performance.

Cardiovascular Exercise:

Examples: Running, cycling, swimming.

Benefits: Improves heart health and circulation, both of which are critical for strong erections.

Strength Training:
Examples: Weight lifting, bodyweight exercises (e.g., squats, lunges).
Benefits: Increases testosterone production, improves muscle tone, and supports hormonal balance.

Pelvic Floor Exercises (Kegels):
Benefits: Strengthens the muscles that support erectile function, improves blood flow to the penis, and enhances orgasm control.

Yoga and Stretching:
Benefits: Reduces stress, improves flexibility, and promotes relaxation, all of which can reduce the risk of ED.

Stress Management and Mental Health
Psychological factors, such as stress, anxiety, and depression, can significantly impact erectile function. Managing stress and improving mental health can help reduce the negative effects of these factors on your sexual performance.

Mindfulness and Meditation:
Practices like mindfulness meditation, deep breathing, and progressive muscle relaxation can

help lower stress levels, improve mood, and enhance focus.

Therapy or Counseling:
If ED is related to psychological issues such as anxiety or past trauma, speaking with a therapist or counselor can be incredibly beneficial. Cognitive Behavioral Therapy (CBT) has been shown to help reduce performance anxiety and improve sexual function.

Relaxation Techniques:
Activities like listening to music, taking a warm bath, or spending time in nature can help reduce stress and promote relaxation.

Adequate Sleep and Hormonal Balance
Poor sleep quality and sleep deprivation can lead to imbalances in hormones like testosterone, which is essential for sexual function. Getting enough quality sleep is crucial for both physical and mental well-being.

Sleep Tips:
Aim for 7-9 hours of sleep per night.
Create a relaxing bedtime routine (e.g., dim the lights, avoid screen time, and practice deep breathing).
Ensure your sleep environment is quiet, dark, and comfortable.

Testosterone and Sleep:
Adequate sleep supports the natural production of testosterone, which plays a key role in libido and erectile health.

Herbal Supplements and Natural Remedies
Certain herbs and supplements have been traditionally used to support erectile health. While they are not a substitute for medical treatment, some may help enhance circulation, balance hormones, and support sexual function.

Ginseng:
Often used in traditional medicine to boost libido, increase energy, and improve blood flow. Studies suggest it may help improve erectile function in some men.

L-arginine:
An amino acid that helps the body produce nitric oxide, which relaxes blood vessels and improves blood flow. It is commonly used as a supplement to support erectile function.

Maca Root:
A Peruvian herb known to boost libido and sexual stamina. Some studies have shown that maca can improve sexual function, particularly in men with mild ED.

Tribulus Terrestris:

A plant that has been shown to increase testosterone levels and improve sexual desire.

Horny Goat Weed (Epimedium):
A traditional herb used to enhance sexual performance by increasing blood flow and improving erectile function.

Yohimbine:
Derived from the bark of the Yohimbe tree, this supplement has been used to treat erectile dysfunction, though it should be taken with caution due to potential side effects.

Maintaining a Healthy Weight
Being overweight or obese can contribute to various health issues, including erectile dysfunction. Excess fat, particularly abdominal fat, can impair circulation, reduce testosterone levels, and lead to other conditions like diabetes and hypertension.

Weight Management Tips:
Focus on a balanced, nutrient-dense diet combined with regular physical activity.
Consider working with a healthcare provider or nutritionist to create a sustainable weight loss plan.

Avoiding Harmful Habits
Certain lifestyle habits can negatively affect erectile health and should be avoided or minimized:

Excessive Alcohol Consumption:
While moderate alcohol intake may not harm erectile function, excessive drinking can impair blood flow and reduce testosterone levels.

Smoking:
Smoking is a major risk factor for cardiovascular disease, which can impair blood flow to the penis. Quitting smoking can significantly improve erectile function.

Recreational Drug Use:
Drugs like cocaine and marijuana can interfere with arousal and erectile function.

Natural remedies and lifestyle changes offer an effective, holistic approach to improving erectile health. By making informed decisions about diet, exercise, stress management, and sleep, you can significantly reduce the risk of erectile dysfunction and enhance sexual performance. While these strategies may take time to show results, they contribute to long-term health improvements that benefit not only sexual function but overall well-being.

CHAPTER 12

Maintaining Sexual Health as You Age

As men age, they often experience changes in sexual health, including a decline in erectile function, libido, and overall sexual satisfaction. While these changes are a normal part of the aging process, many can be managed or even reversed with proactive care, lifestyle adjustments, and the right medical guidance. Maintaining sexual health as you age is not only about addressing erectile dysfunction (ED) but also about fostering overall physical and emotional well-being.

The Impact of Aging on Sexual Health

Decreased Testosterone Levels

Testosterone levels naturally decline with age, starting around the age of 30. Lower levels of this key hormone can lead to reduced libido, erectile dysfunction, and fatigue.

Changes in Erectile Function

As men age, it may take longer to achieve an erection, and the erection may not be as firm or lasting. Blood flow to the penis can decrease due to aging blood vessels and cardiovascular conditions.

Reduced Sexual Desire

Along with physical changes, aging can affect emotional well-being, leading to a decrease in sexual desire or interest. This can also be influenced by stress, anxiety, and depression, which are common in older adults.

Prostate Health
Enlarged prostate or other prostate-related issues can interfere with sexual function and lead to urinary problems, which can affect intimacy.

Strategies for Maintaining Sexual Health as You Age

While aging may bring changes in sexual health, there are many effective ways to counteract these effects and maintain an active, satisfying sex life.

Focus on Cardiovascular Health
Since erectile function is closely tied to blood flow, maintaining a healthy heart and circulatory system is essential for sustaining erections and sexual vitality.

Exercise:
Cardiovascular Activity: Regular aerobic exercise, such as walking, swimming, or cycling, improves circulation and heart health, both critical for erectile function.
Strength Training: Maintaining muscle mass through weight lifting or resistance training also supports metabolic health and testosterone production.

Manage Blood Pressure and Cholesterol:
High blood pressure and high cholesterol can damage blood vessels, impairing blood flow to the penis. Regular monitoring and healthy diet choices can help maintain vascular health.

Maintain a Healthy Weight
Being overweight or obese increases the risk of several health issues that can affect sexual function, including diabetes, high blood pressure, and reduced testosterone levels.

Healthy Diet:
Focus on nutrient-dense foods, including fruits, vegetables, whole grains, and lean proteins. Avoid processed foods, excess sugar, and trans fats, all of which contribute to weight gain and chronic health conditions.

Regular Exercise:
Regular physical activity helps regulate body weight, improve mood, and boost energy levels, which can support sexual function.

Manage Hormonal Health
Hormonal imbalances, particularly low testosterone, are a significant factor in the sexual health of aging men. Understanding and addressing hormonal changes is key to maintaining sexual health as you age.

Testosterone Replacement Therapy (TRT):
If testosterone levels are significantly low, your doctor may recommend TRT, which can improve libido, energy, and erectile function.
Natural Approaches:

Certain lifestyle changes, such as getting enough sleep, reducing stress, and eating a balanced diet, can help optimize testosterone production. Some herbs and supplements like ginseng, maca root, and zinc may also support natural testosterone levels.

Practice Pelvic Floor Exercises
Pelvic floor exercises (such as Kegels) are an excellent way to maintain erectile health and improve sexual function as you age. These exercises strengthen the muscles responsible for sexual performance and urinary control.

Benefits of Kegels for Older Men:
Improved blood flow to the penis.
Enhanced control over erections and ejaculation.
Better urinary control, which can improve confidence and sexual comfort.

How to Perform Kegels:
Contract the muscles used to stop the flow of urine.
Hold for 5 seconds, relax, and repeat for 10-15 reps, 2-3 times per day.

Address Psychological Factors

As men age, psychological factors such as stress, anxiety, depression, and relationship issues can play a significant role in sexual health. Addressing these factors is crucial for maintaining a fulfilling sex life.

Manage Stress and Anxiety:
Practice relaxation techniques like deep breathing, meditation, or yoga to manage stress. Reducing anxiety around sexual performance can lead to better erections and more satisfying experiences.

Relationship Counseling:
If relationship issues are affecting sexual health, consider couples therapy or counseling to improve communication, intimacy, and emotional connection.

Seek Professional Help for Depression:
If depression is affecting your libido and sexual function, working with a therapist or counselor can help you manage your mental health and restore a positive outlook on intimacy.

Sleep and Restorative Health
Sleep plays a critical role in overall health, including hormone production and energy levels. Poor sleep quality can lead to low testosterone, fatigue, and a lack of desire, all of which can negatively impact sexual function.

Aim for 7-9 Hours of Sleep:

Create a sleep-friendly environment by keeping your bedroom dark, quiet, and cool. Avoid screen time before bed and establish a consistent sleep routine.

Restorative Practices:
Engaging in relaxing activities before bed, such as reading, listening to soothing music, or practicing meditation, can improve sleep quality.

Prostate Health

As men age, prostate health can become a significant concern, particularly with conditions such as benign prostatic hyperplasia (BPH) or prostate cancer, which can affect sexual health.

Regular Check-ups:
Regular prostate screenings, including a digital rectal exam (DRE) and prostate-specific antigen (PSA) test, are important for early detection of prostate issues.

Healthy Diet:
Diets rich in fruits, vegetables, and healthy fats (like those found in fish, nuts, and olive oil) are linked to better prostate health. Lycopene-rich foods like tomatoes may also support prostate function.

Stay Hydrated:
Drink plenty of water to support urinary health, as dehydration can worsen prostate symptoms.

Sexual Communication and Experimentation
As relationships mature, sexual needs and desires may evolve. Open communication with your partner about preferences, desires, and intimacy can enhance sexual satisfaction, even as physical changes occur.

Explore New Forms of Intimacy:
Be open to trying new sexual positions, activities, or techniques that are comfortable and enjoyable for both partners.

Mutual Support and Understanding:
Discuss any concerns about aging, sexual performance, or health issues with your partner to foster intimacy and mutual support.

Maintaining sexual health as you age requires a holistic approach that focuses on physical, emotional, and psychological well-being. While aging naturally brings about changes in sexual function, making informed lifestyle choices, addressing health concerns, and maintaining strong relationships can help you continue to enjoy a fulfilling and satisfying sex life. By prioritizing cardiovascular health, managing hormones, exercising regularly, and addressing psychological factors, you can protect your sexual health and maintain vitality well into later years.

CHAPTER 13

Conclusion

Erectile health is an essential component of overall well-being, and while factors like aging, stress, and medical conditions can impact sexual function, there are numerous steps you can take to protect and enhance your erections over time. A holistic approach that integrates physical, emotional, and psychological health is key to maintaining long-term sexual wellness.

Key Steps to Protecting Your Erection

Maintain Cardiovascular Health

Regular exercise, a heart-healthy diet, and effective management of blood pressure, cholesterol, and diabetes are crucial for improving blood flow and preserving erectile function.

Prioritize Diet and Nutrition

Eating a balanced, nutrient-dense diet rich in vitamins, minerals, and antioxidants supports both cardiovascular and hormonal health. Foods that boost circulation, like leafy greens, berries, and omega-3-rich fish, are particularly beneficial for erectile function.

Exercise Regularly

Engage in both aerobic and strength-training exercises to enhance blood flow, regulate hormones, and improve overall stamina. Pelvic floor exercises (Kegels) specifically target the muscles responsible for sexual function and control.

Manage Stress and Mental Health
Psychological factors, including stress, anxiety, and depression, can significantly affect erectile function. Practicing relaxation techniques, seeking therapy if necessary, and maintaining a healthy emotional connection with a partner are crucial for sexual well-being.

Get Quality Sleep
Sleep is vital for hormonal balance and overall health. Prioritize restful, consistent sleep patterns to support testosterone production and prevent sexual health issues.

Monitor and Manage Hormonal Changes
As you age, testosterone levels naturally decline. Staying active, maintaining a healthy weight, and considering testosterone replacement therapy (if appropriate) can help mitigate the effects of lower hormone levels.

Avoid Harmful Habits
Limit alcohol consumption, avoid smoking, and steer clear of recreational drugs. These habits can impair circulation, reduce testosterone, and damage blood

vessels, all of which contribute to erectile dysfunction.

Routine Check-ups and Professional Guidance
Regular check-ups with a healthcare provider ensure early detection of underlying health issues such as cardiovascular disease, diabetes, or prostate problems. Professional guidance is essential in managing ED and preventing long-term complications.

Explore Natural Remedies and Supplements
While not a substitute for medical treatment, certain natural remedies (e.g., ginseng, L-arginine, maca root) can enhance erectile health by improving circulation and hormone balance.

Nurture Your Relationship
Open communication with your partner and exploring new forms of intimacy can maintain sexual satisfaction and emotional connection, which are vital for a fulfilling sex life.

A Long-Term Approach to Sexual Wellness
Protecting your erection and maintaining sexual wellness is not a quick fix; it's a long-term commitment to overall health and well-being. By making consistent, healthy lifestyle choices—such as staying active, managing stress, maintaining a nutritious diet, and prioritizing emotional health—you

can not only protect your erections but also improve the quality of your life in general.

Sexual wellness is intertwined with physical health, emotional balance, and self-care. Fostering these elements together will help ensure that you continue to enjoy a fulfilling and vibrant sex life, no matter your age. Taking a proactive approach now can safeguard your sexual function for years to come, helping you stay confident, satisfied, and healthy.